5

Competency Based Logbook in Microbiology

for Second Professional MBBS

As per the latest CBME Guidelines | Competency Based Undergraduate Curriculum for the Indian Medical Graduate

Name: ______________________________

Roll No.: ______________ University Registration No.: ______________

Date of Admission: ______________________________

Permanent Address: ______________________________

E-mail ID: ______________ Batch: ______________

Mobile No.: ______________________________

5

Competency Based Logbook in Microbiology

for Second Professional MBBS

As per the latest CBME Guidelines | Competency Based Undergraduate Curriculum for the Indian Medical Graduate

Niket Verma MBBS, MD, ACME, FAIMER, MIMSA, MAMS

Assistant Professor
Department of General Medicine
All India Institute of Medical Sciences
Bathinda, Punjab

Poonam Agrawal MBBS, MD, FIMSA, FAHP, ACME

Dean
Maharaja Agrasen Kedar Nath Gupta Medical College and
Maharaja Agrasen Sat Narain Gupta Hospital
Bahadurgarh, Haryana

Megha Maheshwari MD

Professor and Head
Department of Microbiology
Dr Baba Saheb Ambedkar Medical
College and Hospital
New Delhi

CBSPD

CBS Publishers & Distributors Pvt Ltd

New Delhi • Bengaluru • Chennai • Kochi • Kolkata • Lucknow • Mumbai
Gujarat • Hyderabad • Jharkhand • Nagpur • Patna • Pune • Uttarakhand

Disclaimer

Science and technology are constantly changing fields. New research and experience broaden the scope of information and knowledge. The authors have tried their best in giving information available to them while preparing the material for this book. Although all efforts have been made to ensure optimum accuracy of the material, yet it is quite possible some errors might have been left uncorrected. The publisher, the printer, and the authors will not be held responsible for any inadvertent errors or inaccuracies.

Competency Based Logbook in

Microbiology

for Second Professional MBBS

ISBN: 978-93-90709-76-2

First Edition: 2021
Reprint: 2025, **2026**

Published by **Satish Kumar Jain** and produced by **Varun Jain** for
CBS Publishers & Distributors Pvt Ltd
4819/XI Prahlad Street, 24 Ansari Road, Daryaganj, New Delhi 110 002, India
Ph: 011-23289259, 23266838 Website: www.cbspd.com e-mail: delhi@cbspd.com

Corporate Office: 204 FIE, Industrial Area, Patparganj, Delhi 110 092
Ph: 011-4934 4934 Fax: 011-4934 4935 e-mail: publishing@cbspd.com; publicity@cbspd.com

Branches

- **Bengaluru:** Seema House 2975, 17th Cross, KR Road, Banasankari 2nd Stage, Bengaluru 560 070, Karnataka, India
  Ph: +91-80-26771678/79 Fax: +91-80-26771680 e-mail: bangalore@cbspd.com
- **Chennai:** 18/8B, Subbarayan Street, Shenoy Nagar, Chennai 600 030, Tamil Nadu, India
  Ph: +91-44-42032115, 45022115 e-mail: chennai@cbspd.com
- **Kochi:** 42/1325, 1326, Power House Road, Opposite KSEB, 682 018, Kochi, Kerala, India
  Ph: +91-484-4059061-65 e-mail: kochi@cbspd.com
- **Kolkata:** 147, Hind Ceramics Compound, 1st Floor, Nilgunj Road, Belghoria, Kolkata 700 056, West Bengal, India
  Ph: +91-33-25633055-56 e-mail: kolkata@cbspd.com
- **Lucknow:** Basement, Khushnuma Complex, 7-Meerabai Marg (behind Jawahar Bhawan), Lucknow 226 001, UP, India
  Ph: +91-522-4000032 e-mail: tiwari.lucknow@cbspd.com
- **Mumbai:** PWD Shed, Gala No. 25/26, Ramchandra Bhatt Marg, Next to JJ Hospital Gate No. 2
  Opposite Union Bank of India, Noorbaug, Mumbai 400 009, Maharashtra, India
  Ph: +91-22-66661880/89 e-mail: mumbai@cbspd.com

Representatives

- **Gujarat** • **Hyderabad** • **Jharkhand** • **Nagpur** • **Patna** • **Pune** • **Uttarakhand**

For trade terms please contact customercare@cbspd.com

For general enquiries please contact info@cbspd.com

Printed at Chaman Enterprises, Daryaganj, Delhi, India

Preface

This logbook has been designed keeping in mind the requirements of the new Competency Based Medical Education (CBME) curriculum.

Individual departments have the flexibility to decide the list of competencies to be included in this logbook and specify the maximum number of attempts allowed for each activity. Adequate space is provided to enter the details of the competencies and activities, the details of remedial training (if any), the rating for each attempt at the activity and the final decision of the faculty. The assessment scale has only two ratings, 'Scope for further improvement' and 'Satisfactory'; thereby emphasising on positive motivation for all students.

Sections on important topics from the subject have been designed as reflective portfolios with ample space for reflection writing by the student learners. Separate sections have also been designed for SBT (Simulation Based Teaching), AETCOM (Attitude, Ethics and Communication) and Integration.

Introduction

The Competency Based Medical Education (CBME) curriculum for undergraduate medical education was introduced in the academic year 2019–2020. The new curriculum has brought about a fundamental change in the system of medical education in our country. There is greater emphasis on alignment and integration of the various subjects, on the acquisition of specific competencies and essential skills and on the assessment 'for' learning. Maintaining a record of the activities conducted and the competencies and skills acquired is now a mandatory requirement.

This logbook aims to provide a ready format to record the activities, competencies and skills in **Microbiology**. Combined with reflection writing, the records can be used for formative and continuous assessment of the learners as they progress through the year and onwards to Third Professional MBBS. We hope that this logbook will serve as a stimulus to encourage self-directed learning among undergraduate students.

Salient Features

1. Simple tabular format of the templates for recording the activities conducted and competencies and skills acquired
2. An assessment scale with only two ratings, Scope for further improvement and Satisfactory; thereby emphasising on positive motivation for all students
3. Flexibility to record the competencies decided by individual departments
4. Ample space in each row to record and assess all activities under a given competency
5. Reflective portfolios for important topics with encouragement of reflection writing and recording the details of assignments and assessments
6. Separate sections for SBT (Simulation Based Teaching), AETCOM (Attitude, Ethics and Communication) and Integration.

Niket Verma
Poonam Agrawal
Megha Maheshwari

Certificate 1

It is hereby certified that Ms./Mr. ……………………………………………………………, Roll No./University Registration No. ………………………………………………, who is a student of IInd Professional MBBS at………………………………………………………… (name of Medical College), has satisfactorily achieved all competencies (including certifiable competencies) and completed all assignments from Microbiology mentioned in this logbook.

She/He is eligible to appear for the IInd Professional MBBS University examinations in Microbiology which will be conducted by …………………………………………… (name of the affiliating university), from ……………… to……………… .

Signature of Faculty-incharge

Signature of Head of the Department

Signature of Principal/Dean of the College

Certificate 2

It is hereby certified that Ms./Mr. ……………………………………………………………, Roll No./University Registration No. ………………………………………………, who is a student of IInd Professional MBBS at………………………………………………………… (name of Medical College), has NOT achieved all competencies (including certifiable competencies) and/or completed all assignments from Microbiology mentioned in this logbook.

She/He is NOT eligible to appear for the IInd Professional MBBS University examinations in Microbiology which will be conducted by ……………………………… (name of the affiliating university), from ……………… to……………… .

Signature of Faculty-incharge

Signature of Head of the Department

Signature of Principal/Dean of the College

Contents

Section 1: Introduction to Microbiology

Sr. No.	Competency number and description of the activity	Maximum number of attempts allowed for the activity	No. of attempts taken by the learner (with date of each attempt)	Any remedial training needed? (Yes/No) If yes then state the reason(s)	Rating **1.** Scope for further improvement **2.** Satisfactory (All attempts at the activity must be rated separately)	Final decision of faculty **C**– Completed **N**–Not completed	Feedback conveyed by faculty (Yes/No) Signature of faculty (with date)	Feedback received by learner (Yes/No) Signature of learner (with date)
Introduction to Microbiology								
1.								
2.								
3.								
4.								
5.								

Section 1: Introduction to Microbiology

(This page may be used to record the salient points of the discussion as well as any activities, assignments or assessments on the topic)

Sub-topic: Date:

1. Please describe briefly what was discussed OR details of activity/assignment/assessment:

2. What did you learn from the discussion OR the activity/assignment/assessment:

3. Do you feel that the knowledge you have acquired will help you become a better doctor? Please explain in your own words.

Feedback Received (Yes/No):

Section 1A: History and Evolution of Microbiology

(This page may be used to record the salient points of the discussion as well as any activities, assignments or assessments on the topic)

Sub-topic: Date:

1. Please describe briefly what was discussed OR details of activity/assignment/assessment:

2. What did you learn from the discussion OR the activity/assignment/assessment:

3. Do you feel that the knowledge you have acquired will help you become a better doctor? Please explain in your own words.

Feedback Received (Yes/No):

Section 1B: The Role of Microbiology in Disease Diagnosis and Management

(This page may be used to record the salient points of the discussion as well as any activities, assignments or assessments on the topic)

Sub-topic: Date:

1. Please describe briefly what was discussed OR details of activity/assignment/assessment:

2. What did you learn from the discussion OR the activity/assignment/assessment:

3. Do you feel that the knowledge you have acquired will help you become a better doctor? Please explain in your own words.

Feedback Received (Yes/No):

Section 2: General Microbiology

Sr. No.	Competency Number and description of the activity	Maximum number of attempts allowed for the activity	No. of attempts taken by the learner (with date of each attempt)	Any remedial training needed? (Yes/No) If yes then state the reason(s)	Rating **1.** Scope for further improvement **2.** Satisfactory (All attempts at the activity must be rated separately)	Final decision of faculty **C**– Completed **N**–Not completed	Feedback conveyed by faculty (Yes/No) Signature of faculty (with date)	Feedback received by learner (Yes/No) Signature of learner (with date)
General Microbiology								
1.								
2.								
3.								
4.								
5.								

Section 2: General Microbiology

Sr. No.	Competency Number and description of the activity	Maximum number of attempts allowed for the activity	No. of attempts taken by the learner (with date of each attempt)	Any remedial training needed? (Yes/No) If yes then state the reason(s)	Rating **1.** Scope for further improvement **2.** Satisfactory (All attempts at the activity must be rated separately)	Final decision of faculty **C**– Completed **N**–Not completed	Feedback conveyed by faculty (Yes/No) Signature of faculty (with date)	Feedback received by learner (Yes/No) Signature of learner (with date)
General Microbiology								
6.								
7.								
8.								
9.								
10.								

Section 2: General Microbiology

(This page may be used to record the salient points of the discussion as well as any activities, assignments or assessments on the topic)

Sub-topic: Date:

1. Please describe briefly what was discussed OR details of activity/assignment/assessment:

2. What did you learn from the discussion OR the activity/assignment/assessment:

3. Do you feel that the knowledge you have acquired will help you become a better doctor? Please explain in your own words.

Feedback Received (Yes/No):

Section 2A: Causative Agents of Infectious Diseases—Bacteria

(This page may be used to record the salient points of the discussion as well as any activities, assignments or assessments on the topic)

Sub-topic: Date:

1. Please describe briefly what was discussed OR details of activity/assignment/assessment:

2. What did you learn from the discussion OR the activity/assignment/assessment:

3. Do you feel that the knowledge you have acquired will help you become a better doctor? Please explain in your own words.

Feedback Received (Yes/No):

Section 2A: Causative Agents of Infectious Diseases—Bacteria

(This page may be used to record the salient points of the discussion as well as any activities, assignments or assessments on the topic)

Sub-topic: Date:

1. Please describe briefly what was discussed OR details of activity/assignment/assessment:

2. What did you learn from the discussion OR the activity/assignment/assessment:

3. Do you feel that the knowledge you have acquired will help you become a better doctor? Please explain in your own words.

Feedback Received (Yes/No):

Section 2B: Causative Agents of Infectious Diseases—Viruses

(This page may be used to record the salient points of the discussion as well as any activities, assignments or assessments on the topic)

Sub-topic: Date:

1. Please describe briefly what was discussed OR details of activity/assignment/assessment:

2. What did you learn from the discussion OR the activity/assignment/assessment:

3. Do you feel that the knowledge you have acquired will help you become a better doctor? Please explain in your own words.

Feedback Received (Yes/No):

Section 2B: Causative Agents of Infectious Diseases—Viruses

(This page may be used to record the salient points of the discussion as well as any activities, assignments or assessments on the topic)

Sub-topic: Date:

1. Please describe briefly what was discussed OR details of activity/assignment/assessment:

2. What did you learn from the discussion OR the activity/assignment/assessment:

3. Do you feel that the knowledge you have acquired will help you become a better doctor? Please explain in your own words.

Feedback Received (Yes/No):

Section 2C: Causative Agents of Infectious Diseases—Fungi

(This page may be used to record the salient points of the discussion as well as any activities, assignments or assessments on the topic)

Sub-topic: Date:

1. Please describe briefly what was discussed OR details of activity/assignment/assessment:

2. What did you learn from the discussion OR the activity/assignment/assessment:

3. Do you feel that the knowledge you have acquired will help you become a better doctor? Please explain in your own words.

Feedback Received (Yes/No):

Section 2D: Causative Agents of Infectious Diseases—Protozoans

(This page may be used to record the salient points of the discussion as well as any activities, assignments or assessments on the topic)

Sub-topic: Date:

1. Please describe briefly what was discussed OR details of activity/assignment/assessment:

2. What did you learn from the discussion OR the activity/assignment/assessment:

3. Do you feel that the knowledge you have acquired will help you become a better doctor? Please explain in your own words.

Feedback Received (Yes/No):

Section 2D: Causative Agents of Infectious Diseases—Protozoans

(This page may be used to record the salient points of the discussion as well as any activities, assignments or assessments on the topic)

Sub-topic: Date:

1. Please describe briefly what was discussed OR details of activity/assignment/assessment:

2. What did you learn from the discussion OR the activity/assignment/assessment:

3. Do you feel that the knowledge you have acquired will help you become a better doctor? Please explain in your own words.

Feedback Received (Yes/No):

Section 2E: Causative Agents of Infectious Diseases—Helminths

(This page may be used to record the salient points of the discussion as well as any activities, assignments or assessments on the topic)

Sub-topic: Date:

1. Please describe briefly what was discussed OR details of activity/assignment/assessment:

2. What did you learn from the discussion OR the activity/assignment/assessment:

3. Do you feel that the knowledge you have acquired will help you become a better doctor? Please explain in your own words.

Feedback Received (Yes/No):

Section 2E: Causative Agents of Infectious Diseases—Helminths

(This page may be used to record the salient points of the discussion as well as any activities, assignments or assessments on the topic)

Sub-topic: Date:

1. Please describe briefly what was discussed OR details of activity/assignment/assessment:

2. What did you learn from the discussion OR the activity/assignment/assessment:

3. Do you feel that the knowledge you have acquired will help you become a better doctor? Please explain in your own words.

Feedback Received (Yes/No):

Section 2F: Causative Agents of Infectious Diseases—Miscellaneous

(This page may be used to record the salient points of the discussion as well as any activities, assignments or assessments on the topic)

Sub-topic: Date:

1. Please describe briefly what was discussed OR details of activity/assignment/assessment:

2. What did you learn from the discussion OR the activity/assignment/assessment:

3. Do you feel that the knowledge you have acquired will help you become a better doctor? Please explain in your own words.

Feedback Received (Yes/No):

Section 2G: Sample Collection

(This page may be used to record the salient points of the discussion as well as any activities, assignments or assessments on the topic)

Sub-topic: Date:

1. Please describe briefly what was discussed OR details of activity/assignment/assessment:

2. What did you learn from the discussion OR the activity/assignment/assessment:

3. Do you feel that the knowledge you have acquired will help you become a better doctor? Please explain in your own words.

Feedback Received (Yes/No):

Section 2G: Sample Collection

(This page may be used to record the salient points of the discussion as well as any activities, assignments or assessments on the topic)

Sub-topic: Date:

1. Please describe briefly what was discussed OR details of activity/assignment/assessment:

2. What did you learn from the discussion OR the activity/assignment/assessment:

3. Do you feel that the knowledge you have acquired will help you become a better doctor? Please explain in your own words.

Feedback Received (Yes/No):

Section 2H: Culture Media and Culture Methods

Section 2H: Culture Media and Culture Methods

Section 2H: Culture Media and Culture Methods

(This page may be used to record the salient points of the discussion as well as any activities, assignments or assessments on the topic)

Sub-topic: Date:

1. Please describe briefly what was discussed OR details of activity/assignment/assessment:

2. What did you learn from the discussion OR the activity/assignment/assessment:

3. Do you feel that the knowledge you have acquired will help you become a better doctor? Please explain in your own words.

Feedback Received (Yes/No):

Section 2I: Sterilization and Disinfection

Section 2I: Sterilization and Disinfection

Section 2I: Sterilization and Disinfection

(This page may be used to record the salient points of the discussion as well as any activities, assignments or assessments on the topic)

Sub-topic: Date:

1. Please describe briefly what was discussed OR details of activity/assignment/assessment:

2. What did you learn from the discussion OR the activity/assignment/assessment:

3. Do you feel that the knowledge you have acquired will help you become a better doctor? Please explain in your own words.

Feedback Received (Yes/No):

Section 2J: Staining Techniques in Microbiology

Section 2J: Staining Techniques in Microbiology

Section 2J: Staining Techniques in Microbiology

(This page may be used to record the salient points of the discussion as well as any activities, assignments or assessments on the topic)

Sub-topic: Date:

1. Please describe briefly what was discussed OR details of activity/assignment/assessment:

2. What did you learn from the discussion OR the activity/assignment/assessment:

3. Do you feel that the knowledge you have acquired will help you become a better doctor? Please explain in your own words.

Feedback Received (Yes/No):

Section 2K: Microscopy

Section 2K: Microscopy

Section 2K: Microscopy

(This page may be used to record the salient points of the discussion as well as any activities, assignments or assessments on the topic)

Sub-topic: Date:

1. Please describe briefly what was discussed OR details of activity/assignment/assessment:

2. What did you learn from the discussion OR the activity/assignment/assessment:

3. Do you feel that the knowledge you have acquired will help you become a better doctor? Please explain in your own words.

Feedback Received (Yes/No):

Section 2L: Drug Resistance and Monitoring of Antimicrobial Therapy

(This page may be used to record the salient points of the discussion as well as any activities, assignments or assessments on the topic)

Sub-topic: Date:

1. Please describe briefly what was discussed OR details of activity/assignment/assessment:

2. What did you learn from the discussion OR the activity/assignment/assessment:

3. Do you feel that the knowledge you have acquired will help you become a better doctor? Please explain in your own words.

Feedback Received (Yes/No):

Section 2L: Drug Resistance and Monitoring of Antimicrobial Therapy

(This page may be used to record the salient points of the discussion as well as any activities, assignments or assessments on the topic)

Sub-topic: Date:

1. Please describe briefly what was discussed OR details of activity/assignment/assessment:

2. What did you learn from the discussion OR the activity/assignment/assessment:

3. Do you feel that the knowledge you have acquired will help you become a better doctor? Please explain in your own words.

Feedback Received (Yes/No):

Section 2M: Laboratory tests and interpretation of results

Section 2M: Laboratory tests and interpretation of results

Section 2M: Laboratory tests and interpretation of results

(This page may be used to record the salient points of the discussion as well as any activities, assignments or assessments on the topic)

Sub-topic: Date:

1. Please describe briefly what was discussed OR details of activity/assignment/assessment:

2. What did you learn from the discussion OR the activity/assignment/assessment:

3. Do you feel that the knowledge you have acquired will help you become a better doctor? Please explain in your own words.

Feedback Received (Yes/No):

Section 3: Immunology

Sr. No.	Competency Number and description of the activity	Maximum number of attempts allowed for the activity	No. of attempts taken by the learner (with date of each attempt)	Any remedial training needed? (Yes/No) If yes then state the reason(s)	Rating **1.** Scope for further improvement **2.** Satisfactory (All attempts at the activity must be rated separately)	Final decision of faculty **C**– Completed **N**–Not completed	Feedback conveyed by faculty (Yes/No) Signature of faculty (with date)	Feedback received by learner (Yes/No) Signature of learner (with date)
Immunology								
1.								
2.								
3.								
4.								
5.								

Section 3: Immunology

Sr. No.	Competency Number and description of the activity	Maximum number of attempts allowed for the activity	No. of attempts taken by the learner (with date of each attempt)	Any remedial training needed? (Yes/No) If yes then state the reason(s)	Rating **1.** Scope for further improvement **2.** Satisfactory (All attempts at the activity must be rated separately)	Final decision of faculty **C**– Completed **N**–Not completed	Feedback conveyed by faculty (Yes/No) Signature of faculty (with date)	Feedback received by learner (Yes/No) Signature of learner (with date)
Immunology								
6.								
7.								
8.								
9.								
10.								

Section 3: Immunology

(This page may be used to record the salient points of the discussion as well as any activities, assignments or assessments on the topic)

Sub-topic: Date:

1. Please describe briefly what was discussed OR details of activity/assignment/assessment:

2. What did you learn from the discussion OR the activity/assignment/assessment:

3. Do you feel that the knowledge you have acquired will help you become a better doctor? Please explain in your own words.

Feedback Received (Yes/No):

Section 3A: Antigen-Antibody Reactions

Section 3A: Antigen-Antibody Reactions

(This page may be used to record the salient points of the discussion as well as any activities, assignments or assessments on the topic)

Sub-topic: Date:

1. Please describe briefly what was discussed OR details of activity/assignment/assessment:

2. What did you learn from the discussion OR the activity/assignment/assessment:

3. Do you feel that the knowledge you have acquired will help you become a better doctor? Please explain in your own words.

Feedback Received (Yes/No):

Section 3B: Hypersensitivity

Section 3B: Hypersensitivity

(This page may be used to record the salient points of the discussion as well as any activities, assignments or assessments on the topic)

Sub-topic: Date:

1. Please describe briefly what was discussed OR details of activity/assignment/assessment:

2. What did you learn from the discussion OR the activity/assignment/assessment:

3. Do you feel that the knowledge you have acquired will help you become a better doctor? Please explain in your own words.

Feedback Received (Yes/No):

Section 3C: Autoimmunity

(This page may be used to record the salient points of the discussion as well as any activities, assignments or assessments on the topic)

Sub-topic: Date:

1. Please describe briefly what was discussed OR details of activity/assignment/assessment:

2. What did you learn from the discussion OR the activity/assignment/assessment:

3. Do you feel that the knowledge you have acquired will help you become a better doctor? Please explain in your own words.

Feedback Received (Yes/No):

Section 3D: Immunodeficiency

Section 3D: Immunodeficiency

(This page may be used to record the salient points of the discussion as well as any activities, assignments or assessments on the topic)

Sub-topic: Date:

1. Please describe briefly what was discussed OR details of activity/assignment/assessment:

2. What did you learn from the discussion OR the activity/assignment/assessment:

3. Do you feel that the knowledge you have acquired will help you become a better doctor? Please explain in your own words.

Feedback Received (Yes/No):

Section 3E: Transplantation and Tumour Immunity

(This page may be used to record the salient points of the discussion as well as any activities, assignments or assessments on the topic)

Sub-topic: Date:

1. Please describe briefly what was discussed OR details of activity/assignment/assessment:

2. What did you learn from the discussion OR the activity/assignment/assessment:

3. Do you feel that the knowledge you have acquired will help you become a better doctor? Please explain in your own words.

Feedback Received (Yes/No):

Section 3F: Serology

(This page may be used to record the salient points of the discussion as well as any activities, assignments or assessments on the topic)

Sub-topic: Date:

1. Please describe briefly what was discussed OR details of activity/assignment/assessment:

2. What did you learn from the discussion OR the activity/assignment/assessment:

3. Do you feel that the knowledge you have acquired will help you become a better doctor? Please explain in your own words.

Feedback Received (Yes/No):

Section 3G: Immuno-Haematology

(This page may be used to record the salient points of the discussion as well as any activities, assignments or assessments on the topic)

Sub-topic: Date:

1. Please describe briefly what was discussed OR details of activity/assignment/assessment:

2. What did you learn from the discussion OR the activity/assignment/assessment:

3. Do you feel that the knowledge you have acquired will help you become a better doctor? Please explain in your own words.

Feedback Received (Yes/No):

Section 3H: Vaccines

Section 3H: Vaccines

(This page may be used to record the salient points of the discussion as well as any activities, assignments or assessments on the topic)

Sub-topic: Date:

1. Please describe briefly what was discussed OR details of activity/assignment/assessment:

2. What did you learn from the discussion OR the activity/assignment/assessment:

3. Do you feel that the knowledge you have acquired will help you become a better doctor? Please explain in your own words.

Feedback Received (Yes/No):

Section 4: Systemic Microbiology

Section 4A: Cardiovascular System

Sr. No.	Competency Number and description of the activity	Maximum number of attempts allowed for the activity	No. of attempts taken by the learner (with date of each attempt)	Any remedial training needed? (Yes/No) If yes then state the reason(s)	Rating **1.** Scope for further improvement **2.** Satisfactory (All attempts at the activity must be rated separately)	Final decision of faculty **C**– Completed **N**–Not completed	Feedback conveyed by faculty (Yes/No) Signature of faculty (with date)	Feedback received by learner (Yes/No) Signature of learner (with date)
Cardiovascular System								
1.								
2.								
3.								
4.								
5.								

Section 4B: Respiratory System

Sr. No.	Competency Number and description of the activity	Maximum number of attempts allowed for the activity	No. of attempts taken by the learner (with date of each attempt)	Any remedial training needed? (Yes/No) If yes then state the reason(s)	Rating **1.** Scope for further improvement **2.** Satisfactory (All attempts at the activity must be rated separately)	Final decision of faculty **C**– Completed **N**–Not completed	Feedback conveyed by faculty (Yes/No) Signature of faculty (with date)	Feedback received by learner (Yes/No) Signature of learner (with date)
Respiratory System								
1.								
2.								
3.								
4.								
5.								

Section 4C: Gastrointestinal System

Sr. No.	Competency Number and description of the activity	Maximum number of attempts allowed for the activity	No. of attempts taken by the learner (with date of each attempt)	Any remedial training needed? (Yes/No) If yes then state the reason(s)	Rating **1.** Scope for further improvement **2.** Satisfactory (All attempts at the activity must be rated separately)	Final decision of faculty **C**– Completed **N**–Not completed	Feedback conveyed by faculty (Yes/No) Signature of faculty (with date)	Feedback received by learner (Yes/No) Signature of learner (with date)
Gastrointestinal System								
1.								
2.								
3.								
4.								
5.								

Section 4D: Hepatobiliary System

Sr. No.	*Competency Number and description of the activity*	*Maximum number of attempts allowed for the activity*	*No. of attempts taken by the learner (with date of each attempt)*	*Any remedial training needed? (Yes/No) If yes then state the reason(s)*	*Rating* **1.** *Scope for further improvement* **2.** *Satisfactory (All attempts at the activity must be rated separately)*	*Final decision of faculty* **C–** *Completed* **N**–*Not completed*	*Feedback conveyed by faculty (Yes/No) Signature of faculty (with date)*	*Feedback received by learner (Yes/No) Signature of learner (with date)*
Hepatobiliary System								
1.								
2.								
3.								
4.								
5.								

Section 4E: Blood

Sr. No.	Competency Number and description of the activity	Maximum number of attempts allowed for the activity	No. of attempts taken by the learner (with date of each attempt)	Any remedial training needed? (Yes/No) If yes then state the reason(s)	Rating **1.** Scope for further improvement **2.** Satisfactory (All attempts at the activity must be rated separately)	Final decision of faculty **C**– Completed **N**–Not completed	Feedback conveyed by faculty (Yes/No) Signature of faculty (with date)	Feedback received by learner (Yes/No) Signature of learner (with date)
Blood								
1.								
2.								
3.								
4.								
5.								

Section 4F: Nervous System

Sr. No.	*Competency Number and description of the activity*	*Maximum number of attempts allowed for the activity*	*No. of attempts taken by the learner (with date of each attempt)*	*Any remedial training needed? (Yes/No) If yes then state the reason(s)*	*Rating* **1.** *Scope for further improvement* **2.** *Satisfactory (All attempts at the activity must be rated separately)*	*Final decision of faculty* **C–** *Completed* **N**–*Not completed*	*Feedback conveyed by faculty (Yes/No) Signature of faculty (with date)*	*Feedback received by learner (Yes/No) Signature of learner (with date)*
Nervous System								
1.								
2.								
3.								
4.								
5.								

Section 4G: Genitourinary System

Sr. No.	*Competency Number and description of the activity*	*Maximum number of attempts allowed for the activity*	*No. of attempts taken by the learner (with date of each attempt)*	*Any remedial training needed? (Yes/No) If yes then state the reason(s)*	*Rating* **1.** *Scope for further improvement* **2.** *Satisfactory (All attempts at the activity must be rated separately)*	*Final decision of faculty* **C**– *Completed* **N**–*Not completed*	*Feedback conveyed by faculty (Yes/No) Signature of faculty (with date)*	*Feedback received by learner (Yes/No) Signature of learner (with date)*
Genitourinary System								
1.								
2.								
3.								
4.								
5.								

Section 4H: Musculoskeletal System

Sr. No.	*Competency Number and description of the activity*	*Maximum number of attempts allowed for the activity*	*No. of attempts taken by the learner (with date of each attempt)*	*Any remedial training needed? (Yes/No) If yes then state the reason(s)*	*Rating* **1.** *Scope for further improvement* **2.** *Satisfactory (All attempts at the activity must be rated separately)*	*Final decision of faculty* **C–** *Completed* **N**–*Not completed*	*Feedback conveyed by faculty (Yes/No) Signature of faculty (with date)*	*Feedback received by learner (Yes/No) Signature of learner (with date)*
Musculoskeletal System								
1.								
2.								
3.								
4.								
5.								

Section 4I: Skin and Soft Tissue

Sr. No.	Competency Number and description of the activity	Maximum number of attempts allowed for the activity	No. of attempts taken by the learner (with date of each attempt)	Any remedial training needed? (Yes/No) If yes then state the reason(s)	Rating **1.** Scope for further improvement **2.** Satisfactory (All attempts at the activity must be rated separately)	Final decision of faculty **C–** Completed **N**–Not completed	Feedback conveyed by faculty (Yes/No) Signature of faculty (with date)	Feedback received by learner (Yes/No) Signature of learner (with date)
Skin and Soft Tissue								
1.								
2.								
3.								
4.								
5.								

Section 4J: Miscellaneous

Sr. No.	*Competency Number and description of the activity*	*Maximum number of attempts allowed for the activity*	*No. of attempts taken by the learner (with date of each attempt)*	*Any remedial training needed? (Yes/No) If yes then state the reason(s)*	*Rating* **1.** *Scope for further improvement* **2.** *Satisfactory (All attempts at the activity must be rated separately)*	*Final decision of faculty* **C**– *Completed* **N**–*Not completed*	*Feedback conveyed by faculty (Yes/No) Signature of faculty (with date)*	*Feedback received by learner (Yes/No) Signature of learner (with date)*
Miscellaneous								
1.								
2.								
3.								
4.								
5.								

Section 4: Systemic Microbiology

(This page may be used to record the salient points of the discussion as well as any activities, assignments or assessments on the topic)

Sub-topic: Date:

1. Please describe briefly what was discussed OR details of activity/assignment/assessment:

2. What did you learn from the discussion OR the activity/assignment/assessment:

3. Do you feel that the knowledge you have acquired will help you become a better doctor? Please explain in your own words.

Feedback Received (Yes/No):

Section 5: Miscellaneous Topics

Section 5A: Zoonoses

Sr. No.	Competency Number and description of the activity	Maximum number of attempts allowed for the activity	No. of attempts taken by the learner (with date of each attempt)	Any remedial training needed? (Yes/No) If yes then state the reason(s)	Rating **1.** Scope for further improvement **2.** Satisfactory (All attempts at the activity must be rated separately)	Final decision of faculty **C**– Completed **N**–Not completed	Feedback conveyed by faculty (Yes/No) Signature of faculty (with date)	Feedback received by learner (Yes/No) Signature of learner (with date)
Zoonoses								
1.								
2.								
3.								
4.								
5.								

Section 5B: Opportunistic Infections

Sr. No.	*Competency Number and description of the activity*	*Maximum number of attempts allowed for the activity*	*No. of attempts taken by the learner (with date of each attempt)*	*Any remedial training needed? (Yes/No) If yes then state the reason(s)*	*Rating* **1.** *Scope for further improvement* **2.** *Satisfactory (All attempts at the activity must be rated separately)*	*Final decision of faculty* **C–** *Completed* **N**–*Not completed*	*Feedback conveyed by faculty (Yes/No) Signature of faculty (with date)*	*Feedback received by learner (Yes/No) Signature of learner (with date)*
Opportunistic Infections								
1.								
2.								
3.								
4.								
5.								

Section 5C: Healthcare Associated Infections

Sr. No.	Competency Number and description of the activity	Maximum number of attempts allowed for the activity	No. of attempts taken by the learner (with date of each attempt)	Any remedial training needed? (Yes/No) If yes then state the reason(s)	Rating **1.** Scope for further improvement **2.** Satisfactory (All attempts at the activity must be rated separately)	Final decision of faculty **C**– Completed **N**–Not completed	Feedback conveyed by faculty (Yes/No) Signature of faculty (with date)	Feedback received by learner (Yes/No) Signature of learner (with date)
Healthcare Associated Infections								
1.								
2.								
3.								
4.								
5.								

Section 5D: Emerging Infectious Diseases

Sr. No.	*Competency Number and description of the activity*	*Maximum number of attempts allowed for the activity*	*No. of attempts taken by the learner (with date of each attempt)*	*Any remedial training needed? (Yes/No) If yes then state the reason(s)*	*Rating* **1.** *Scope for further improvement* **2.** *Satisfactory (All attempts at the activity must be rated separately)*	*Final decision of faculty* **C**– *Completed* **N**–*Not completed*	*Feedback conveyed by faculty (Yes/No) Signature of faculty (with date)*	*Feedback received by learner (Yes/No) Signature of learner (with date)*
Emerging Infectious Diseases								
1.								
2.								
3.								
4.								
5.								

Section 5E: Infection Control Practices

Sr. No.	Competency Number and description of the activity	Maximum number of attempts allowed for the activity	No. of attempts taken by the learner (with date of each attempt)	Any remedial training needed? (Yes/No) If yes then state the reason(s)	Rating **1.** Scope for further improvement **2.** Satisfactory (All attempts at the activity must be rated separately)	Final decision of faculty **C**– Completed **N**–Not completed	Feedback conveyed by faculty (Yes/No) Signature of faculty (with date)	Feedback received by learner (Yes/No) Signature of learner (with date)
Infection Control Practices								
1.								
2.								
3.								
4.								
5.								

Section 5F: Personal Protective Equipment

Sr. No.	*Competency Number and description of the activity*	*Maximum number of attempts allowed for the activity*	*No. of attempts taken by the learner (with date of each attempt)*	*Any remedial training needed? (Yes/No) If yes then state the reason(s)*	*Rating* **1.** *Scope for further improvement* **2.** *Satisfactory (All attempts at the activity must be rated separately)*	*Final decision of faculty* **C–** *Completed* **N**–*Not completed*	*Feedback conveyed by faculty (Yes/No) Signature of faculty (with date)*	*Feedback received by learner (Yes/No) Signature of learner (with date)*
Personal Protective Equipment								
1.								
2.								
3.								
4.								
5.								

Section 5A: Zoonoses

(This page may be used to record the salient points of the discussion as well as any activities, assignments or assessments on the topic)

Sub-topic: Date:

1. Please describe briefly what was discussed OR details of activity/assignment/assessment:

2. What did you learn from the discussion OR the activity/assignment/assessment:

3. Do you feel that the knowledge you have acquired will help you become a better doctor? Please explain in your own words.

Feedback Received (Yes/No):

Section 5B: Opportunistic Infections

(This page may be used to record the salient points of the discussion as well as any activities, assignments or assessments on the topic)

Sub-topic: Date:

1. Please describe briefly what was discussed OR details of activity/assignment/assessment:

2. What did you learn from the discussion OR the activity/assignment/assessment:

3. Do you feel that the knowledge you have acquired will help you become a better doctor? Please explain in your own words.

Feedback Received (Yes/No):

Section 5C: Healthcare Associated Infections

Section 5C: Healthcare Associated Infections

(This page may be used to record the salient points of the discussion as well as any activities, assignments or assessments on the topic)

Sub-topic: Date:

1. Please describe briefly what was discussed OR details of activity/assignment/assessment:

2. What did you learn from the discussion OR the activity/assignment/assessment:

3. Do you feel that the knowledge you have acquired will help you become a better doctor? Please explain in your own words.

Feedback Received (Yes/No):

Section 5D: Emerging Infectious Diseases

Section 5D: Emerging Infectious Diseases

(This page may be used to record the salient points of the discussion as well as any activities, assignments or assessments on the topic)

Sub-topic: Date:

1. Please describe briefly what was discussed OR details of activity/assignment/assessment:

2. What did you learn from the discussion OR the activity/assignment/assessment:

3. Do you feel that the knowledge you have acquired will help you become a better doctor? Please explain in your own words.

Feedback Received (Yes/No):

Section 5E: Infection Control Practices

Section 5E: Infection Control Practices

(This page may be used to record the salient points of the discussion as well as any activities, assignments or assessments on the topic)

Sub-topic: Date:

1. Please describe briefly what was discussed OR details of activity/assignment/assessment:

2. What did you learn from the discussion OR the activity/assignment/assessment:

3. Do you feel that the knowledge you have acquired will help you become a better doctor? Please explain in your own words.

Feedback Received (Yes/No):

Section 5F: Personal Protective Equipment

Section 5F: Personal Protective Equipment

(This page may be used to record the salient points of the discussion as well as any activities, assignments or assessments on the topic)

Sub-topic: Date:

1. Please describe briefly what was discussed OR details of activity/assignment/assessment:

2. What did you learn from the discussion OR the activity/assignment/assessment:

3. Do you feel that the knowledge you have acquired will help you become a better doctor? Please explain in your own words.

Feedback Received (Yes/No):

Section 6: Recent Advances in Microbiology

Section 6: Recent Advances in Microbiology

(This page may be used to record the salient points of the discussion as well as any activities, assignments or assessments on the topic)

Sub-topic: Date:

1. Please describe briefly what was discussed OR details of activity/assignment/assessment:

2. What did you learn from the discussion OR the activity/assignment/assessment:

3. Do you feel that the knowledge you have acquired will help you become a better doctor? Please explain in your own words.

Feedback Received (Yes/No):

Section 7: Simulation Based Teaching (Skills Lab)

(This page may be used to record the salient points of the discussion as well as any activities, assignments or assessments on the topic)

Sub-topic: Date:

1. Please describe briefly what was discussed OR details of activity/assignment/assessment:

2. What did you learn from the discussion OR the activity/assignment/assessment:

3. Do you feel that the knowledge you have acquired will help you become a better doctor? Please explain in your own words.

Feedback Received (Yes/No):

Section 7: Simulation Based Teaching (Skills Lab)

(This page may be used to record the salient points of the discussion as well as any activities, assignments or assessments on the topic)

Sub-topic: Date:

1. Please describe briefly what was discussed OR details of activity/assignment/assessment:

2. What did you learn from the discussion OR the activity/assignment/assessment:

3. Do you feel that the knowledge you have acquired will help you become a better doctor? Please explain in your own words.

Feedback Received (Yes/No):

Section 7: Simulation Based Teaching (Skills Lab)

(This page may be used to record the salient points of the discussion as well as any activities, assignments or assessments on the topic)

Sub-topic: Date:

1. Please describe briefly what was discussed OR details of activity/assignment/assessment:

2. What did you learn from the discussion OR the activity/assignment/assessment:

3. Do you feel that the knowledge you have acquired will help you become a better doctor? Please explain in your own words.

Feedback Received (Yes/No):

Section 7: Simulation Based Teaching (Skills Lab)

(This page may be used to record the salient points of the discussion as well as any activities, assignments or assessments on the topic)

Sub-topic: Date:

1. Please describe briefly what was discussed OR details of activity/assignment/assessment:

2. What did you learn from the discussion OR the activity/assignment/assessment:

3. Do you feel that the knowledge you have acquired will help you become a better doctor? Please explain in your own words.

Feedback Received (Yes/No):

Section 8: Attitude, Ethics and Communication (AETCOM)

Sr. No.	*Competency Number and description of the activity*	*Maximum number of attempts allowed for the activity*	*No. of attempts taken by the learner (with date of each attempt)*	*Any remedial training needed? (Yes/No) If yes then state the reason(s)*	*Rating* **1.** *Scope for further improvement* **2.** *Satisfactory (All attempts at the activity must be rated separately)*	*Final decision of faculty* **C–** *Completed* **N**–*Not completed*	*Feedback conveyed by faculty (Yes/No) Signature of faculty (with date)*	*Feedback received by learner (Yes/No) Signature of learner (with date)*
Attitude, Ethics and Communication (AETCOM)								
1.								
2.								
3.								
4.								
5.								

Section 8: Attitude, Ethics and Communication (AETCOM)

(This page may be used to record the salient points of the discussion as well as any activities, assignments or assessments on the topic)

Sub-topic:

Date:

1. Please describe briefly what was discussed OR details of activity/assignment/assessment:

2. What did you learn from the discussion OR the activity/assignment/assessment:

3. Do you feel that the knowledge you have acquired will help you become a better doctor? Please explain in your own words.

Feedback Received (Yes/No):

Section 8: Attitude, Ethics and Communication (AETCOM)

(This page may be used to record the salient points of the discussion as well as any activities, assignments or assessments on the topic)

Sub-topic: Date:

1. Please describe briefly what was discussed OR details of activity/assignment/assessment:

2. What did you learn from the discussion OR the activity/assignment/assessment:

3. Do you feel that the knowledge you have acquired will help you become a better doctor? Please explain in your own words.

Feedback Received (Yes/No):

Section 9: Integration

Sr. No.	Competency Number and description of the activity	Maximum number of attempts allowed for the activity	No. of attempts taken by the learner (with date of each attempt)	Any remedial training needed? (Yes/No) If yes then state the reason(s)	Rating **1.** Scope for further improvement **2.** Satisfactory (All attempts at the activity must be rated separately)	Final decision of faculty **C**– Completed **N**–Not completed	Feedback conveyed by faculty (Yes/No) Signature of faculty (with date)	Feedback received by learner (Yes/No) Signature of learner (with date)
Integration								
1.								
2.								
3.								
4.								
5.								

Section 9: Integration

Sr. No.	Competency Number and description of the activity	Maximum number of attempts allowed for the activity	No. of attempts taken by the learner (with date of each attempt)	Any remedial training needed? (Yes/No) If yes then state the reason(s)	Rating **1.** Scope for further improvement **2.** Satisfactory (All attempts at the activity must be rated separately)	Final decision of faculty **C**– Completed **N**–Not completed	Feedback conveyed by faculty (Yes/No) Signature of faculty (with date)	Feedback received by learner (Yes/No) Signature of learner (with date)
Integration								
6.								
7.								
8.								
9.								
10.								

Section 9: Integration

(This page may be used to record the salient points of the discussion as well as any activities, assignments or assessments on the topic)

Sub-topic: Date:

1. Please describe briefly what was discussed OR details of activity/assignment/assessment:

2. What did you learn from the discussion OR the activity/assignment/assessment:

3. Do you feel that the knowledge you have acquired will help you become a better doctor? Please explain in your own words.

Feedback Received (Yes/No):

Final Summary

Sr. No.	Section	Dates (dd/mm/yy)	Overall assessment (complete/incomplete	Signature of the faculty-incharge/HoD (with date)
Introduction to Microbiology				
A	History and Evolution of Microbiology			
B	The Role of Microbiology in Disease Diagnosis and Management			
General Microbiology				
A	Causative Agents of Infectious Diseases—Bacteria			
B	Causative Agents of Infectious Diseases—Viruses			
C	Causative Agents of Infectious Diseases—Fungi			
D	Causative Agents of Infectious Diseases—Protozoans			
E	Causative Agents of Infectious Diseases—Helminths			
F	Causative Agents of Infectious Diseases—Miscellaneous			
G	Sample Collection			
H	Culture Media and Culture Methods			
I	Sterilization and Disinfection			

Final Summary

Sr. No.	Section	Dates (dd/mm/yy)	Overall assessment (complete/incomplete	Signature of the faculty-incharge/HoD (with date)
	General Microbiology			
J	Staining Techniques in Microbiology			
K	Microscopy			
L	Drug Resistance and Monitoring of Antimicrobial Therapy			
M	Laboratory Tests and Interpretation of Results			
	Immunology			
A	Antigen-antibody Reactions			
B	Hypersensitivity			
C	Autoimmunity			
D	Immunodeficiency			
E	Transplantation and Tumour Immunity			
F	Serology			
G	Immuno-Haematology			
H	Vaccines			

Final Summary

Sr. No.	Section	Dates (dd/mm/yy)	Overall assessment (complete/incomplete	Signature of the faculty-incharge/HoD (with date)
	Systemic Microbiology			
A	Cardiovascular System			
B	Respiratory System			
C	Gastrointestinal System			
D	Hepatobiliary System			
E	Blood			
F	Nervous System			
G	Genitourinary System			
H	Musculoskeletal System			
I	Skin and Soft Tissue			
J	Miscellaneous			
	Miscellaneous Topics			
A	Zoonoses			
B	Opportunistic Infections			

Final Summary

Sr. No.	Section	Dates (dd/mm/yy)	Overall assessment (complete/incomplete	Signature of the faculty-incharge/HoD (with date)
Miscellaneous Topics				
C	Healthcare Associated Infections			
D	Emerging Infectious Diseases			
E	Infection Control Practices			
F	Personal Protective Equipment			
Recent Advances in Microbiology				
Simulation Based Teaching (Skills Lab)				
Attitude, Ethics and Communication (AETCOM)				
Integration				